42 Powerful Cancer Preventing Juice Recipes:

Naturally Recovery and Prevent Cancer by Increasing Specific Vitamins and Minerals Your Body Needs to Fight Back

By

Joe Correa CSN

COPYRIGHT

This publication is designed to provide accurate and authoritative information in regard to the subject matter covered. It is sold with the understanding that neither the author nor the publisher is engaged in rendering medical advice. If medical advice or assistance is needed, consult with a doctor. This book is considered a guide and should not be used in any way detrimental to your health. Consult with a physician before starting this nutritional plan to make sure it's right for you.

ACKNOWLEDGEMENTS

This book is dedicated to my friends and family that have had mild or serious illnesses so that you may find a solution and make the necessary changes in your life.

42 Powerful Cancer Preventing Juice Recipes:

Naturally Recovery and Prevent Cancer by Increasing Specific Vitamins and Minerals Your Body Needs to Fight Back

By

Joe Correa CSN

CONTENTS

ABOUT THE AUTHOR

After years of Research, I honestly believe in the positive effects that proper nutrition can have over the body and mind. My knowledge and experience has helped me live healthier throughout the years and which I have shared with family and friends. The more you know about eating and drinking healthier, the sooner you will want to change your life and eating habits.

Nutrition is a key part in the process of being healthy and living longer so get started today. The first step is the most important and the most significant.

INTRODUCTION

42 Powerful Cancer Preventing Juice Recipes: Naturally Recovery and Prevent Cancer by Increasing Specific Vitamins and Minerals Your Body Needs to Fight Back

By Joe Correa CSN

About 10-12 million people get cancer every year which makes cancer one of the leading causes of death in the modern world. In the past couple of decades, cancer has escalated to epidemic proportions and affects nearly one out of two men and one out of three women. With 7-8 million lives taken each year due to this disease, I can definitely say that preventing cancer should be your number one priority.

Some statistics say that breast cancer in women and lung cancer in men are two of the most common types of cancer in the world.

One of the major causes for this disease is our modern lifestyles which surround us with different toxins, cancerous substances, and stress. But the main reason is probably poor nutrition for most people. The lack of basic nutrients weakens our immune system which leads to serious and long-term damage to your health and eventually becomes cancer. Most food is full of artificial flavors, colors, additives, stabilizers, and preservatives. Although some of these substances are harmless, many of them are extremely toxic and can deprive our organism of some important nutrients. Although most people know these facts, in theory, they can't seem to find enough time to plan their meals on a daily basis, which is why fast food has become so popular.

This is exactly why juicing should be your number one choice in preventing and fighting cancer. It requires almost no time at all but provides you with an amazing amount of nutrients your body needs in order to build up the immune system and reduce the possibility of cancer. These cancer preventing juice recipes are designed to give you exactly that, all the important nutrients in just a couple of minutes. Try them and see what a difference they can make in your life!

42 POWERFUL CANCER PREVENTING JUICE RECIPES: NATURALLY RECOVERY AND PREVENT CANCER BY INCREASING SPECIFIC VITAMINS AND MINERALS YOUR BODY NEEDS TO FIGHT BACK

1.   Sweet Potato Carrot Juice

Ingredients:

2 large carrots

1 small sweet potato, peeled

2 medium-sized green apples, cored

1 large orange, peeled

¼ tsp of pumpkin pie spice

Preparation:

Combine all ingredients except pumpkin pie spice in a juicer and process until juiced.

Transfer the juice to serving glasses and add few ice cubes.

Sprinkle with some pumpkin pie spice and serve.

Nutritional information per serving: Kcal: 147, Protein: 2.1g, Carbs: 35.4g, Fats: 0.1g

2.   Ginger Chia Juice

Ingredients:

3 large carrots

2 large apples, cored

½ tsp of ginger, ground

1 tbsp of chia seeds

Preparation:

Combine all ingredients except chia seeds in a juicer and process until juiced.

Transfer to serving glasses and add few ice cubes. Sprinkle with chia seeds before serving for extra nutrients. Enjoy!

Nutritional information per serving: Kcal: 177, Protein: 3.2g, Carbs: 28.4g, Fats: 4.6g

3. Kale Squash Juice

Ingredients:

¼ cup of fresh kale

½ yellow squash, peeled

1 medium-sized broccoli

1 large apple, cored

¼ cup of fresh spinach

4 small carrots

Preparation:

Combine all ingredients in a juicer and process until juiced.

Transfer to serving glasses and add few ice cubes. Serve immediately.

Nutritional information per serving: Kcal: 81, Protein: 2.3g, Carbs: 18.4g, Fats: 0.2g

4.   Watermelon Juice

Ingredients:

1 cup of watermelon, peeled and seeded

1 cup of pineapple, peeled

½ large lemon, peeled

½ tsp of ginger, ground

Preparation:

Combine all ingredients in a juicer and process until juiced.

Transfer to serving glasses and add few ice cubes. Serve immediately!

Nutritional information per serving: Kcal: 41, Protein: 1.4g, Carbs: 10.2g, Fats: 0.1g

5.　　Cancun Juice

Ingredients:

½ cup of fresh kale

1 large lime, peeled

1 large cucumber

1 celery stalk

1 small jalapeno pepper, seeded

Preparation:

Combine all ingredients in a juicer and process until juiced. Add coconut water if it is too spicy.

Transfer to serving glasses and add a few ice cubes.

Serve immediately.

Nutritional information per serving: Kcal: 171, Protein: 3.2g, Carbs: 47.3g, Fats: 1.3g

6.   Flaxseed Brown Juice

Ingredients:

2 large carrots

½ cup of fresh spinach

2 tbsp of fresh parsley

2 large apples, cored

¼ tsp of ginger, ground

1 tbsp of flaxseeds

Preparation:

Combine all ingredients in a juicer except flaxseeds. Process until juiced.

Transfer to serving glasses and add few ice cubes.

Sprinkle with flaxseeds and serve!

Nutritional information per serving: Kcal: 119, Protein: 4.3g, Carbs: 62.2g, Fats: 2.3g

7.   Lemon Kale Juice

Ingredients:

½ cup of fresh kale

1 lemon, peeled

2 large green apples, cored

1 large pear, cored

Preparation:

Combine all ingredients in a juicer and process until juiced.

Transfer to serving glasses and add few ice cubes before serving.

Enjoy!

Nutritional information per serving: Kcal: 120, Protein: 3.2g, Carbs: 62.5g, Fats: 1.2g

8.   Broccoli Juice

Ingredients:

1 cup of broccoli

2 large oranges, peeled

1 large cucumber, peeled

1 large carrot

Preparation:

Combine all ingredients in a juicer and process until juiced.

Transfer to serving glasses and add few ice cubes.

Serve immediately!

Nutritional information per serving: Kcal: 68, Protein: 2.3g, Carbs: 19.7g, Fats: 0.1g

9.   Collard Green Juice

Ingredients:

½ cup of collard greens

½ tsp of ginger, ground

1 large cucumber

¼ cup of fresh parsley

1 large apple, cored

Preparation:

Combine all ingredients in a juicer and process until juiced.

Transfer to serving glasses and add few ice cubes.

Serve immediately.

Nutritional information per serving: Kcal: 96, Protein: 3.1g, Carbs: 28.7g, Fats: 1.2g

10. Fennel Tangerine Juice

Ingredients:

1 large fennel

½ cup of fresh kale

1 large green apple, cored

4 tangerines, peeled

Preparation:

Place all ingredients in a juicer and process until juiced.

Transfer to serving glasses and add few ice cubes or refrigerate before use.

Nutritional information per serving: Kcal: 121, Protein: 4.3g, Carbs: 31.3g, Fats: 1.3g

11. Green Grape Juice

Ingredients:

1 cup of green grapes

2 large cucumbers

1 large pear, cored

1 lime, peeled

Preparation:

Combine all ingredients in a juicer and process until juiced.

Transfer to serving glasses and refrigerate for 30 minutes before serving.

Nutritional information per serving: Kcal: 113, Protein: 18.3g, Carbs: 31.3g, Fats: 0.1g

12.   Watercress Juice

Ingredients:

½ cup of watercress

2 large green apples, cored

1 large lemon, peeled

1 large lime, peeled

Preparation:

Combine all ingredients except chia seeds in a juicer and process until juiced.

Transfer to serving glasses and add few ice cubes.

Serve immediately.

Nutritional information per serving: Kcal: 101, Protein: 17.2g, Carbs: 28.8g, Fats: 0.2g

13. Pineapple Cantaloupe Juice

Ingredients:

1 cup of cantaloupe, peeled

½ pineapple, peeled

2 large green apples, cored

½ cup of fresh kale

Preparation:

Combine all ingredients in a juicer and process until juiced.

Transfer to serving glasses and add few ice cubes, or refrigerate for 30 minutes before serving.

Nutritional information per serving: Kcal: 115, Protein: 1.2g, Carbs: 28.8g, Fats: 1.2g

14.   Radish Fennel Juice

Ingredients:

6 medium-sized radishes

1 small fennel

1 large orange, peeled

5 large celery stalks

1 large cucumber

Preparation:

Combine all ingredients in a juicer and process until juiced.

Transfer to serving glasses and refrigerate for a while before serving.

Nutritional information per serving: Kcal: 110, Protein: 6.1g, Carbs: 28.7g, Fats: 1.2g

15.　Swiss Chard Basil Juice

Ingredients:

½ cup of Swiss chard

½ cup of fresh basil

1 large lime, peeled

2 large green apples, cored

¼ cup of fresh mint

Preparation:

Combine all ingredients in a juicer and process until juiced.

Transfer to serving glasses and add few ice cubes or refrigerate until use.

Nutritional information per serving: Kcal: 114, Protein: 2.3g, Carbs: 30.4g, Fats: 0.2g

16.   Green Cabbage Juice

Ingredients:

½ cup of green cabbage

4 celery stalks

1 large green apple, cored

3 large carrots

1 large lemon, peeled

1 tbsp of liquid honey

Preparation:

Combine all ingredients in a juicer and process until juiced.

Transfer to serving glasses and refrigerate for 20 minutes before serving.

Nutritional information per serving: Kcal: 162, Protein: 3.1g, Carbs: 39.3g, Fats: 0.1g

17.   Grapefruit Rosemary Juice

Ingredients:

3 large grapefruits, peeled

3 large oranges, peeled

1 large lemon, peeled

½ tsp of fresh rosemary

Preparation:

Combine all ingredients in a juicer and process until juiced.

Transfer to serving glasses and add few ice cubes.

Sprinkle with fresh rosemary and serve immediately!

Nutritional information per serving: Kcal: 140, Protein: 3.4g, Carbs: 37.6g, Fats: 0.1g

18. Strawberry Peach Juice

Ingredients:

3 large peaches, pitted

1 cup of strawberries

1 large green apple, cored

¼ tsp of ginger, ground

Preparation:

Combine all ingredients in a juicer and process until juiced.

Transfer to serving glasses and add few ice cubes, or refrigerate for 1 hour before serving.

Nutritional information per serving: Kcal: 64, Protein: 1.2g, Carbs: 18.3g, Fats: 0.1g

19.   Cilantro Juice

Ingredients:

½ cup of cilantro

3 celery stalks

1 large green apple, cored

1 large lemon, peeled

½ tsp of ginger, ground

Preparation:

Combine all ingredients except ginger in a juicer.

Process until juiced and transfer to serving glasses and stir in the ginger.

Add few ice cubes and serve immediately.

Nutritional information per serving: Kcal: 73, Protein: 2.2g, Carbs: 26.7g, Fats: 0.1g

20.   Pomegranate Kale Juice

Ingredients:

½ cup of pomegranate seeds

½ cup of fresh kale

1 large green apple, cored

¼ tsp of ginger, ground

3-4 fresh mint leaves

Preparation:

Combine pomegranate seeds, kale, mint, and apple in a juicer and process until juiced.

Transfer to serving glasses and stir in the ginger and some extra pomegranate seeds if you like.

Add few ice cubes and serve immediately.

Nutritional information per serving: Kcal: 143, Protein: 6.2g, Carbs: 41.2g, Fats: 2.4g

21.   Tomato Garlic Juice

Ingredients:

2 large tomatoes, halved

2 garlic cloves, peeled

3 large cucumbers

1 large bell pepper, seeded

1 small shallot

1 large lime, peeled

¼ cup of fresh cilantro

Preparation:

Combine all ingredients in a juicer and process until juiced.

Transfer to serving glasses and add few ice cubes or refrigerate for a while before serving.

Nutritional information per serving: Kcal: 109, Protein: 6.4g, Carbs: 38.5g, Fats: 1.2g

22.   Pineapple Carrot Juice

Ingredients:

1 cup of pineapple, peeled

2 large carrots

½ cup of watercress

1 large lemon, peeled

¼ tsp of ginger root

Preparation:

Combine all ingredients in a juicer and process until juiced.

Transfer to serving glasses and enjoy!

Nutritional information per serving: Kcal: 101, Protein: 3.1g, Carbs: 34.2g, Fats: 1.1g

23.   Strawberry Kiwi Juice

Ingredients:

2 kiwis, peeled

1 large cucumber

1 cup of fresh strawberries

1 small lime, peeled

2 tbsp of fresh mint

Preparation:

Combine all ingredients in a juicer and process until juiced.

Transfer to serving glasses and refrigerate for a while until use.

Nutritional information per serving: Kcal: 91, Protein: 3.1g, Carbs: 29.9g, Fats: 0.9g

24.   Apple Chia Juice

Ingredients:

1 large red apple, cored

1 large lemon, peeled

1 large bell pepper, seeded

3 tbsp of chia seeds

Preparation:

Combine apple, lemon, and bell pepper and run trough juicer.

Process until juiced and stir in the chia seeds.

Let it stand for 15 minutes to thicken and stir well before use.

Nutritional information per serving: Kcal: 135, Protein: 4.2g, Carbs: 31.3g, Fats: 6.2g

25. Spicy Grapefruit Juice

Ingredients:

1 large kiwi, peeled

½ medium-sized grapefruit, peeled

1 large lemon, peeled

3 celery stalks

¼ tsp of ginger, ground

¼ tsp of Cayenne pepper, ground

A handful of watercress

Preparation:

Combine kiwi, grapefruit, lemon, celery, and watercress in a juicer and process until juiced.

Transfer to serving glasses and stir in the ginger and cayenne pepper.

Enjoy!

Nutritional information per serving: Kcal: 61, Protein: 2.1g, Carbs: 20.4g, Fats: 1.1g

26.   Turmeric Cucumber Juice

Ingredients:

1 large cucumber

1 cup of pineapple, chopped

3 celery stalks

½ cup of fresh spinach

¼ tsp of ginger, ground

¼ tsp of turmeric, ground

Preparation:

Combine all ingredients except ginger and turmeric in a juicer.

Process until juiced and transfer to serving glasses. Stir in the turmeric and ginger and serve.

Nutritional information per serving: Kcal: 109, Protein: 3.3g, Carbs: 61.2g, Fats: 1.3g

27.   Zucchini Roma Juice

Ingredients:

2 medium-sized zucchini

1 garlic clove, peeled

6 asparagus stalks

3 Roma tomatoes

4 large carrots

Preparation:

Combine all ingredients in a juicer and process until juiced.

Transfer to serving glasses and enjoy immediately.

Nutritional information per serving: Kcal: 92, Protein: 5.4g, Carbs: 27.3g, Fats: 0.9g

28.   Cinnamon Chia Juice

Ingredients:

1 tbsp of chia seeds

1 large apple, cored

1 cup of fresh spinach

¼ tsp of cinnamon, ground

Preparation:

Combine apple and spinach in a juicer and process until juiced.

Transfer to serving glasses and stir in the cinnamon and chia seeds.

Set aside for 20 minutes to thicken, then serve.

Nutritional information per serving: Kcal: 121, Protein: 4.3g, Carbs: 27.8g, Fats: 5.3g

29. Green Coconut Juice

Ingredients:

1 large lime, peeled

3 oz of coconut water

5 small celery stalks

¼ cup od fresh mint

¼ cup of fresh spinach

Preparation:

Combine lime, celery, spinach, and mint in a juicer and process until juiced.

Transfer to serving glasses and stir in coconut water. Refrigerate for 20 minutes before use.

Nutritional information per serving: Kcal: 45, Protein: 2.2g, Carbs: 16.8g, Fats: 1.6g

30.   Cauliflower Broccoli Juice

Ingredients:

2 cups of cauliflower, chopped

1 cup of fresh broccoli

4 large carrots

1 large green apple, cored

1 tsp of ginger root

Preparation:

Combine all ingredients in a juicer and process until juiced.

Transfer to serving glasses and garnish with mint or add ice cubes for refreshment.

Enjoy!

Nutritional information per serving: Kcal: 136, Protein: 6.3g, Carbs: 42.8g, Fats: 1.2g

31. Ice Green Juice

Ingredients:

1 medium-sized cucumber

1 large pear, cored

3 large carrots

1 large lemon, peeled

¼ cup of fresh mint

½ cup of broccoli

1 tsp of ginger root

½ tsp of green tea powder

2 oz of water

Preparation:

Combine cucumber, pear, carrots, lemon, mint, ginger, and broccoli in a juicer and process until juiced.

Mix water with green tea in a serving glasses and add juice.

Mix with a spoon and add few ice cubes. Serve immediately.

Nutritional information per serving: Kcal: 141, Protein: 5.5g, Carbs: 45.7g, Fats: 0.9g

32.   Orange Green Juice

Ingredients:

2 large oranges, peeled

½ cup of fresh broccoli, chopped

3 large carrots

4 collard green leaves

4 fresh kale leaves

1 garlic clove, peeled

Preparation:

Combine all ingredients in a juicer and process until juiced.

Transfer to serving glasses and serve immediately.

Nutritional information per serving: Kcal: 171, Protein: 9.2g, Carbs: 43.3g, Fats: 2.3g

33. Orange Honey Juice

Ingredients:

2 large oranges, peeled

½ cup of grapefruit, chopped

3-4 fresh kale leaves

1 tsp of liquid honey

¼ tsp of ginger, ground

Preparation:

Combine oranges, grapefruit, and kale in a juicer and process until juiced.

Transfer to serving glasses and stir in the honey and ginger.

Serve immediately.

Nutritional information per serving: Kcal: 128, Protein: 7.3g, Carbs: 34.5g, Fats: 1.1g

34.　Sweet Potato Ginger Juice

Ingredients:

2 medium-sized sweet potatoes, peeled

1 large peach, pitted and halved

¼ tsp of ginger, ground

¼ tsp of cinnamon, ground

Preparation:

Combine potatoes and peach in a juicer and process until juiced.

Transfer to serving glasses and stir in the ginger and cinnamon.

Serve immediately.

Nutritional information per serving: Kcal: 159, Protein: 5.2g, Carbs: 50.1g, Fats: 0.9g

35. Strawberry Tomato Juice

Ingredients:

1 cup of fresh strawberries

2 large tomatoes

2 large carrots

1 large orange, peeled

1 large bell pepper, seeded

Preparation:

Combine all ingredients in a juicer and process until juiced.

Transfer to serving glasses and refrigerate for 30 minutes before serving.

Nutritional information per serving: Kcal: 104, Protein: 3.9g, Carbs: 31.2g, Fats: 1.1g

36. Orange Turmeric Juice

Ingredients:

1 large orange bell pepper, seeded

1 large orange, peeled

1 large carrot

1 large lemon, peeled

1 small cucumber

¼ tsp of turmeric, ground

Preparation:

Combine all ingredients except turmeric in a juicer and process until juiced.

Transfer to serving glasses and stir in the turmeric. Serve immediately.

Nutritional information per serving: Kcal: 152, Protein: 4.2g, Carbs: 48.1g, Fats: 1.3g

37.   Arugula Juice

Ingredients:

1 cup of fresh arugula

1 large lemon, peeled

1 large lime, peeled

1 large orange, peeled

1 large kiwi, peeled

1 small cucumber

Preparation:

Combine all ingredients in a juicer and process until juiced.

Transfer to serving glasses and serve immediately.

Nutritional information per serving: Kcal: 192, Protein: 3.1g, Carbs: 31.6g, Fats: 0.9g

38.   Mango Juice

Ingredients:

1 large mango, peeled

1 large cucumber

½ cup of fresh spinach

2 oz of coconut, grated

Preparation:

Combine mango, cucumber, and spinach in a juicer and process until juiced.

Transfer to serving glasses and stir in the grated coconut.

Refrigerate for 1 hour before serving.

Nutritional information per serving: Kcal: 68, Protein: 1.9g, Carbs: 20.1g, Fats: 0.5g

39.   Bok Choy Leek Juice

Ingredients:

1 medium-sized leek

1 small baby bok choy

¼ cup of fresh basil

1 large green apple, cored

2 large carrots

4-5 fresh kale leaves

Preparation:

Combine all ingredients in a juicer and process until juiced.

Transfer to serving glasses and refrigerate before use.

Nutritional information per serving: Kcal: 169, Protein: 2.3g, Carbs: 46.2g, Fats: 1.9g

40.   Strawberry Kale Juice

Ingredients:

2 cups of fresh strawberries

1 large green apple, cored

1 large cucumber

4-5 fresh kale leaves

Preparation:

Combine all ingredients in a juicer and process until juiced.

Transfer to serving glasses and serve immediately.

Nutritional information per serving: Kcal: 184, Protein: 7.7g, Carbs: 49.5g, Fats: 2.1g

41.   Thai Cantaloupe Juice

Ingredients:

1 cup of cantaloupe, peeled

1 small Romaine lettuce head

1 tbsp of coconut, grated

½ cup of fresh basil

1 large cucumber

Preparation:

Combine all ingredients in a juicer and process until juiced.

Transfer to serving glasses and serve immediately.

Nutritional information per serving: Kcal: 112, Protein: 2.3g, Carbs: 22.6g, Fats: 1.1g

42.   Ginger Beet Juice

Ingredients:

2 large beets, trimmed

1 large cucumber

1 large red apple, cored

1 large lime, peeled

¼ tsp of ginger, ground

Preparation:

Combine all ingredients except ginger in a juicer and process until juiced.

Transfer to serving glasses and stir in the ginger. Refrigerate for 1 hour before serving.

Nutritional information per serving: Kcal: 109, Protein: 2.8g, Carbs: 33.6g, Fats: 0.7g

ADDITIONAL TITLES FROM THIS AUTHOR

70 Effective Meal Recipes to Prevent and Solve Being Overweight: Burn Fat Fast by Using Proper Dieting and Smart Nutrition

By

Joe Correa CSN

48 Acne Solving Meal Recipes: The Fast and Natural Path to Fixing Your Acne Problems in Less Than 10 Days!

By

Joe Correa CSN

41 Alzheimer's Preventing Meal Recipes: Reduce or Eliminate Your Alzheimer's Condition in 30 Days or Less!

By

Joe Correa CSN

70 Effective Breast Cancer Meal Recipes: Prevent and Fight Breast Cancer with Smart Nutrition and Powerful Foods

By

Joe Correa CSN